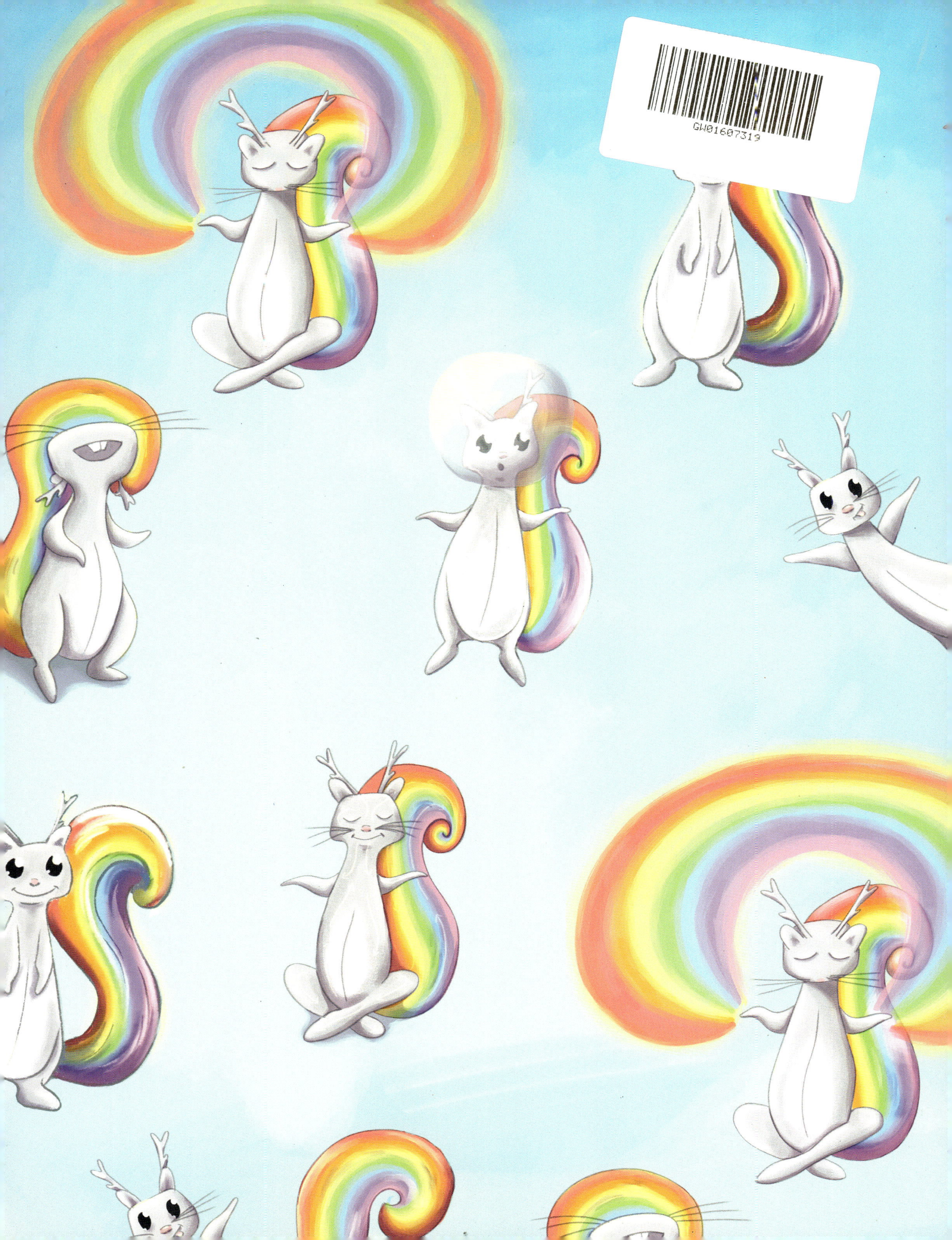
GW01607319

My dear Hugo,

I wrote this story for you, I hope when I am long gone you will remember the times Dad and I sat and read these pages with you.
I like to think of all the precious moments that will be created with this book, the love, calmness and peace.
These tools can help to build a brighter future for our upcoming heroes (future generations).

All our love

MAM & DAd

ISBN 978-1-8383091-0-7

www.bhaktihealing.ie

A Time for Us

Liz Reilly

Corryn Webb

Introduction for adult:

We are living in a fast-paced world with little time to relax. Sometimes, it can be difficult to even know how to relax. It isn't just us adults who are experiencing this, children are too. I believe it is vital that young children are given the tools they need to cope with the fast-paced society we are living in. With so much pressure and stress put upon the shoulders of ourselves and our children, it's more important than ever to find time to unwind, relax and slow down the pace of life. But first, we need to learn how to do so. This book aims to give you the tools as an adult to show the child ways to do just that. With short and gentle exercises, this book will guide you both through a mindful, healing journey, which will provide you and your child with an enriching time together.

I currently work as a reiki practitioner and yoga teacher. I am also a mother of a child with additional needs. The insights I have gained through both my work and my son, have inspired me to help others. I would love to share some of my energy and knowledge with you throughout this book. The good news is you don't need to have a host of qualifications to be able to learn how to find inner harmony; if you follow my exercises carefully, you will be able to replicate them yourself. I hope to help create inner harmony with each reader, who in turn will create harmony and peace everywhere they go.

Each part of this book guides you through the energy points in the body. These energy points are known as the Chakra System and are explained more in the table on page 11. They are in the 'subtle body'. The subtle body describes the various layers of vibrating energy that make up a human being beyond the obvious physical layer. Each chakra stores every moment and every emotion from birth. Remember, energy can never be destroyed - only redirected. We are trillions of energy cells caught up in this beautiful skin suit.

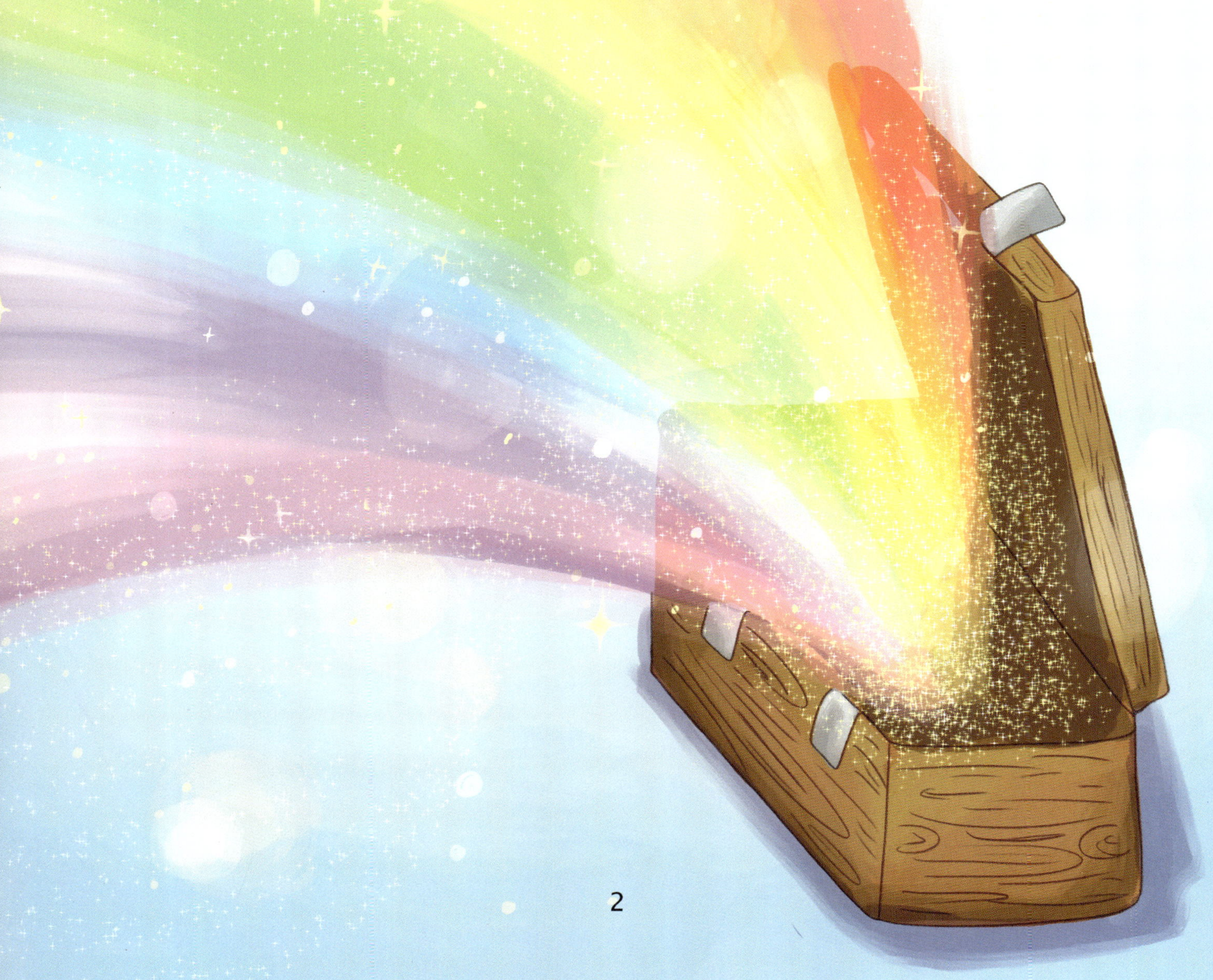

Sometimes, our energy can become blocked, underactive or overactive. When we create time and space to connect within, it can assist in keeping our energy flowing smoothly and a sense of peace within. We all feed off each other's energy. This book will allow you and your child to connect, slow down and become more centred.

As you work your way through these pages, you will become calm and, in turn, your listener will also become calm. It is up to you which order you work through the exercises, although I always recommend starting with exercise 1 first and then choosing which to do next depending upon what is most appropriate. Use the index to decide which section is the most appropriate for your child's current emotional state. How many you do at a time is also up to you; you may feel like you only have time for one, you may feel like it's important to work through several of the exercises in one session. Whatever you wish to do is OK, use this book how you feel it best works for you and your child.

If you or your listener are new to mindfulness or imagery work, you may find it difficult to adjust to at first or you may find it a little uncomfortable. Don't worry, everything new can be a bit odd at the start, and that's OK. Give it time, give it patience, give it perseverance and you will soon find that it becomes easier and feels a more natural process.

Within the exercises, you will see a lot of emphasis on deep breathing, this takes the body into a parasympathetic state, which helps it to relax and slows the heart rate down. It also promotes a healthy gut - a lot of research states that the gut is the 'second brain' and a vital player in the body's immune system. Healthy gut, healthy mind. You will also notice that within the exercises there are some blanks. These are there for you and/or your child to fill in using your imaginations. You will be amazed how quickly you will fill in the blanks and how differently you do so each time you carry out the same exercise.

You and your listener deserve this time together.

I have an incredible son, Hugo, who has taught me a huge amount. This book was inspired by him; Hugo was diagnosed with Autism Spectrum Disorder when he was 3 years old. I wanted to equip him with the tools he needs to help him throughout his whole life – not just whilst being a child, but into adulthood too. Learning mindful practises now can make a huge difference to the future – for us all. When I began mindfulness practices with Hugo, I saw some subtle changes in him which made a big difference to everyday life. Hugo is a lot calmer in new environments since I have started mindfulness with him. It made me realise how important it is, not just for my own son or for those with atypical neurological development, but for everyone to have the ability to relax, be calm and centre themselves. I decided I had to help others and so the process of writing began.

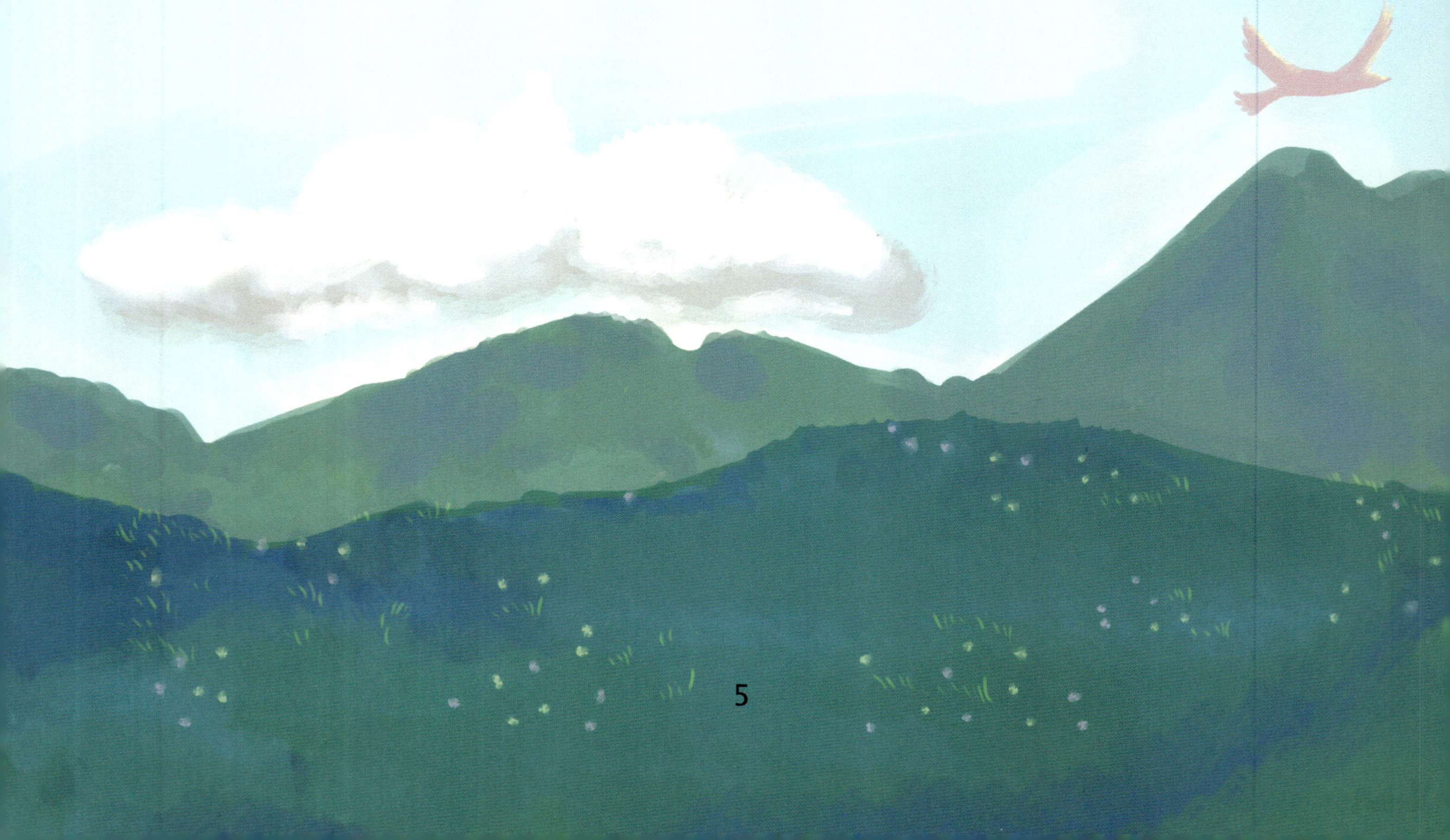

The tools a child (and yourself!) can learn whilst carrying out the activities within this book can help in a wide variety of situations - from being anxious when starting school, to taking a driving test, to being involved in a conflict. Providing children with tools now, will help them forever.
Hugo may be a warrior child now, but one day he will be a grown man.

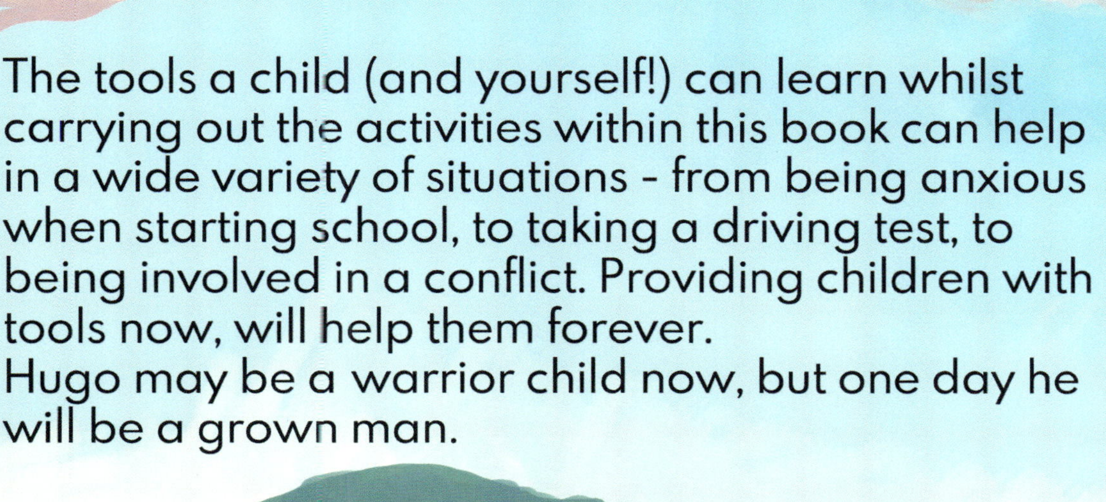

Namaste,
(I honour the light that shines in me and that also shines within you)
Liz

Introduction for child

I hope you are ready for a great adventure with your reader. I know some days can be very busy with lots of homework or having to go to lots of places. It's nice to just sit and be sometimes. I wrote this book just for you; I hope you like it.

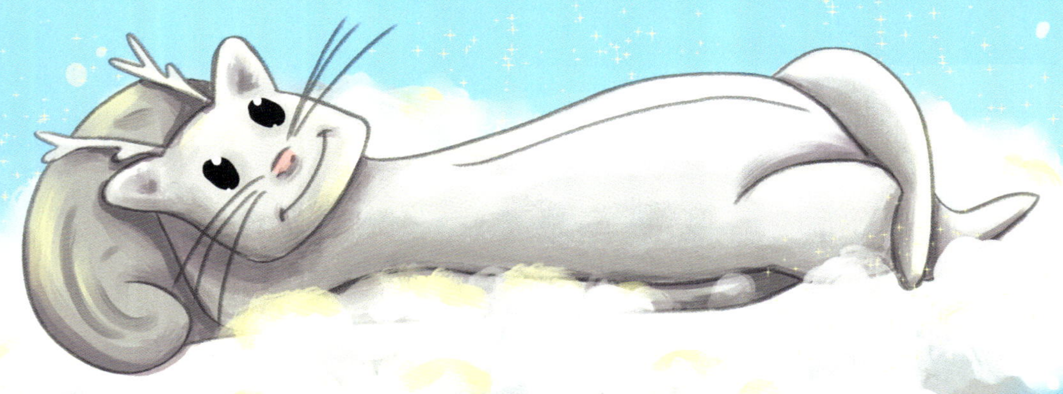

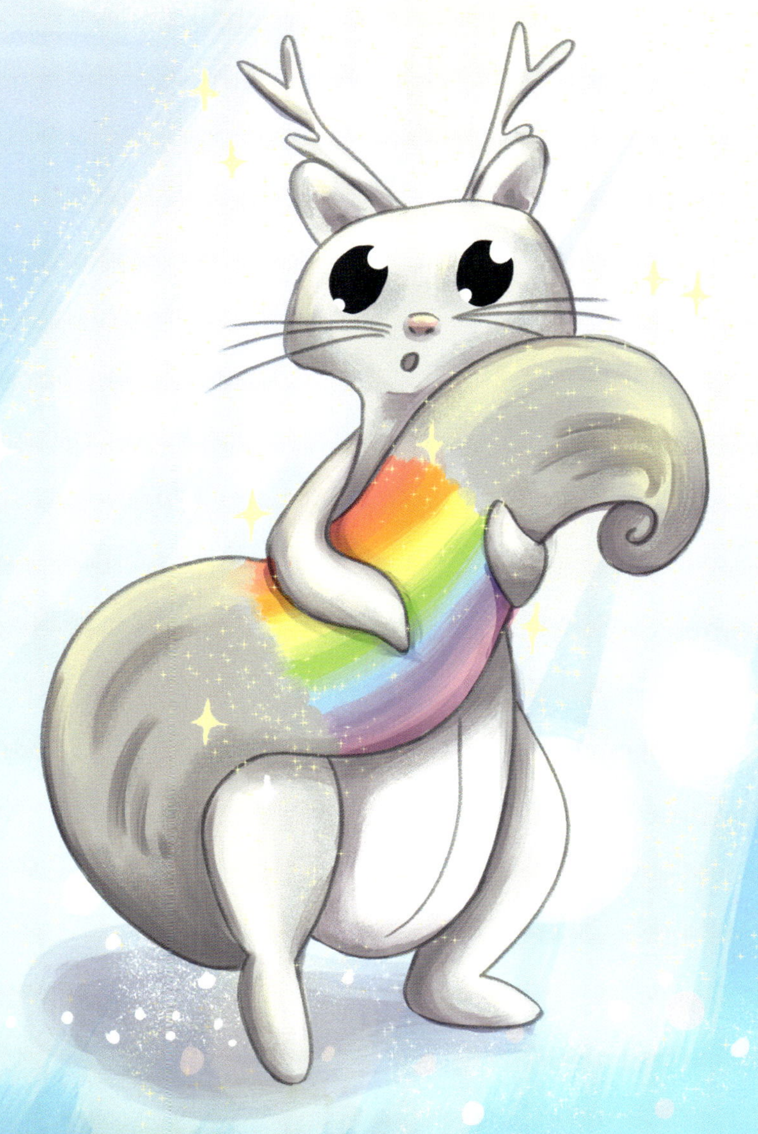

Did you know that there is a magical rainbow inside you? YES, a rainbow! Seven beautiful colours. Red, orange, yellow, green, blue, indigo and violet. Sometimes, the colours aren't vibrant and shiny, they get a little dull when we are tired or worried or sad. But don't worry if you think your rainbow isn't very shiny, I can help you make that rainbow really sparkle!

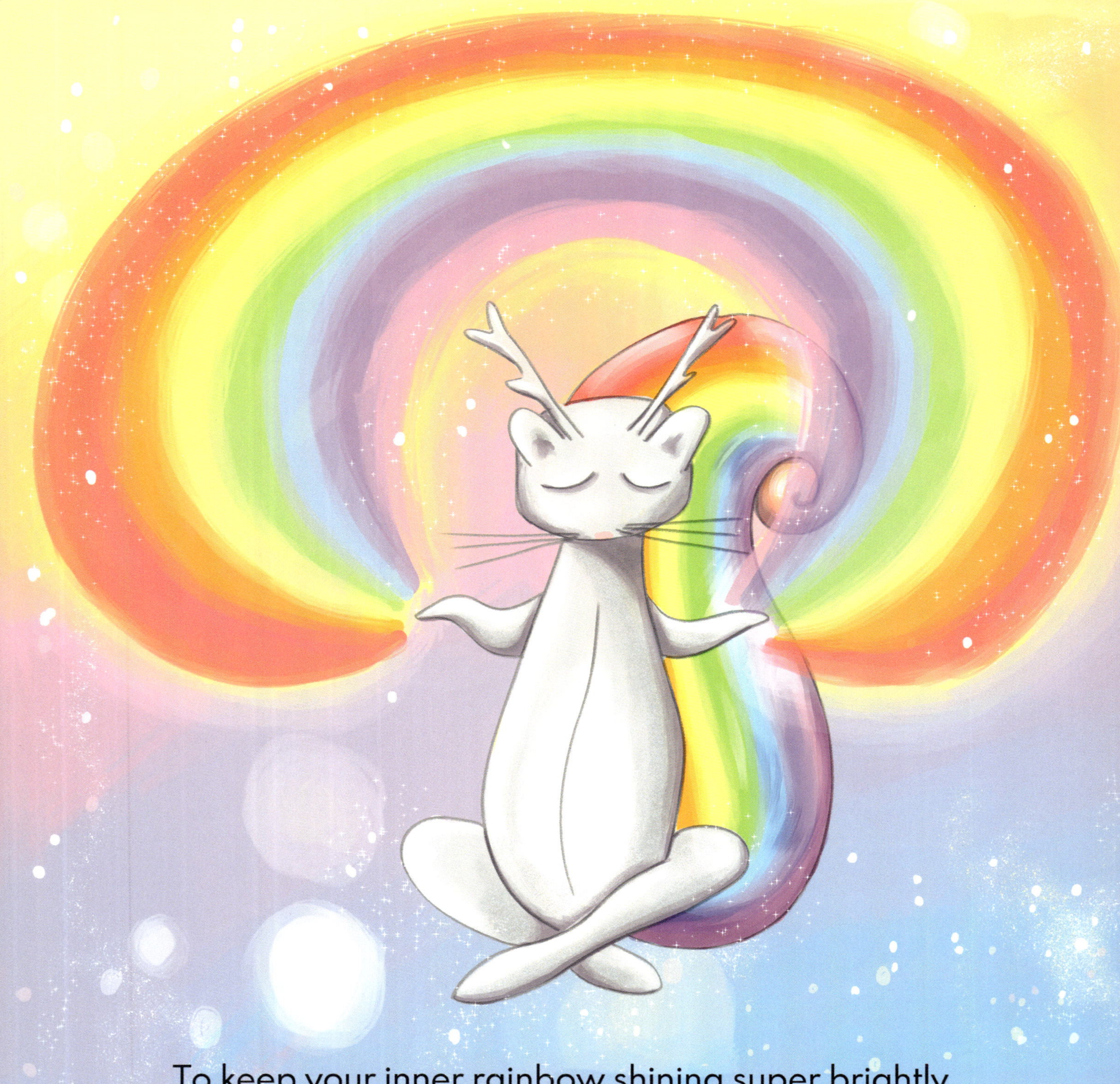

To keep your inner rainbow shining super brightly, there are wonderful things you can do with your reader in this book. You will soon learn that you find ways to make your rainbow shine when you are at school or with friends or anywhere if you feel you need them, and you won't need a reader with you to help you. Your rainbow will be as bright as ever because of you!

After you read this book, it will be like the wind came and blew away the clouds and you will sparkle from the inside out.
Have lots of fun,

All my love,

Liz

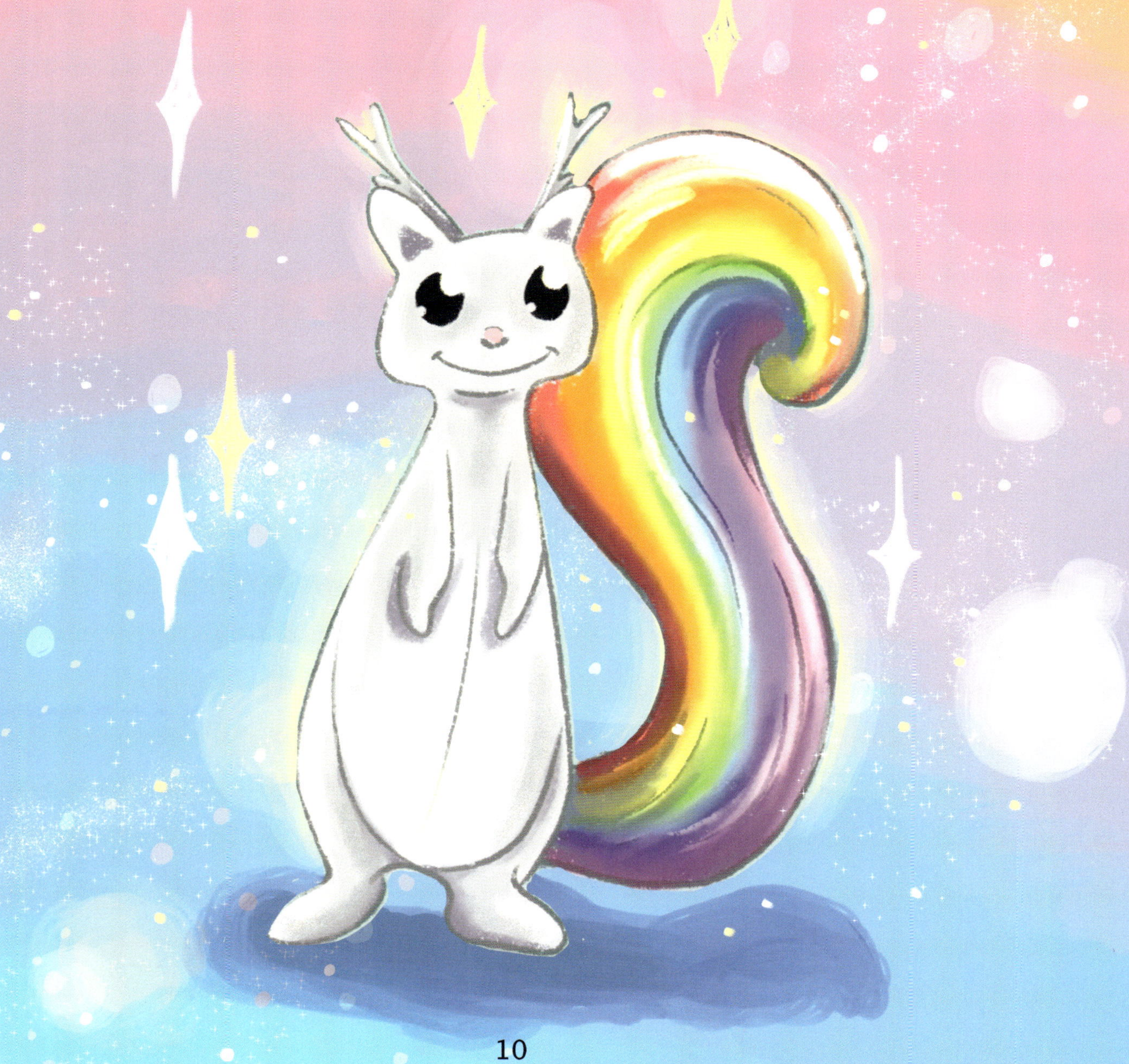

Section	Title	Chakra	Colour	Promotes
1	Grounding	Root Chakra	Red for Root	**Root Chakra:** Promotes a sense of safe and secure
2	Heart to Head	Heart and Crown Chakra	Green for Heart White for Crown	**Heart Chakra:** Promotes giving and love. Crown Chakra is to source/ unlimited
3	Communication	Throat Chakra	Blue for Throat	**Throat Chakra:** Helps with barriers, and feelings such as
4	Emotions	Heart and Sacral Chakra	Green for Heart Orange for Sacral	**Heart Chakra:** Helps with love/ all levels. Sacral Chakra of creativity and
5	Tummy Love	Solar Plexus	Yellow for Solar Plexus	**Solar Plexus:** Helps with power and
6	Magical Journey	Sacral Chakra	Orange for Sacral	**Sacral Chakra:** The seat of and expression
7	Red Cave	Root Chakra	Red for Root	**Root Chakra:** Responsible for feeling safe. It promotes a connection when

	Use when	Affirmations
feeling	You or the child feel uncentred or have an inability to focus or concentrate	I am safe I am powerful I believe in me I am secure
receiving our connection energy	You or the child have any sadness or overthinking. On a physical level this would be good for headaches	I am loved / I am happy I am kind to myself I am open to all the abundance of the universe
communication shyness	You or the child are having difficulty with expressing emotions	I am honest / I trust myself I speak my truth I can express myself with ease
emotions on is the seat emotions	You or the child need help in regulating your emotions	I am happy with life I am feeling complete peace / I trust my feelings
self-confidence, innerstrength	You or the child are feeling worried or anxious or struggling with self-worth and needing empowerment	I stand in my power I am worthy / I am strong I can do anything that I desire
creativity	You or the child feel stressed or struggling to express yourselves	I am complete / I accept all my emotions / I feel clear and free / I am all that I need
stable and sense of balanced	You or the child feel the need to connect with others and think of the wider world	I am safe / I am centred I am confident in all I do I have all I need

Grounding

This time is just for you and me. Let's both close our eyes and take a few deep breaths together. Feel your belly fill up like a balloon when you breathe in.
When you breathe out, imagine you are blowing a big bubble. Let's give our breath a colour.
Mine is ____ today.
What colour is yours?

With each deep breath we take, let's imagine that the colour of our breath starts to flow all around our body. See it now, flowing into your head, neck, arms, your heart, tummy and legs. It's flowing out of our feet and into the ground like the roots of a big tree. See the tree in your mind. Its beautiful thick trunk and all the lovely leaves.

Do you know that trees help us to breathe fresh, clean air? We need to look after all the beautiful trees on Earth. They are also home to lots of lovely birds. Can you sing like a bird?

Close your eyes, let's try and listen to all the sounds around us?
Can you hear any?

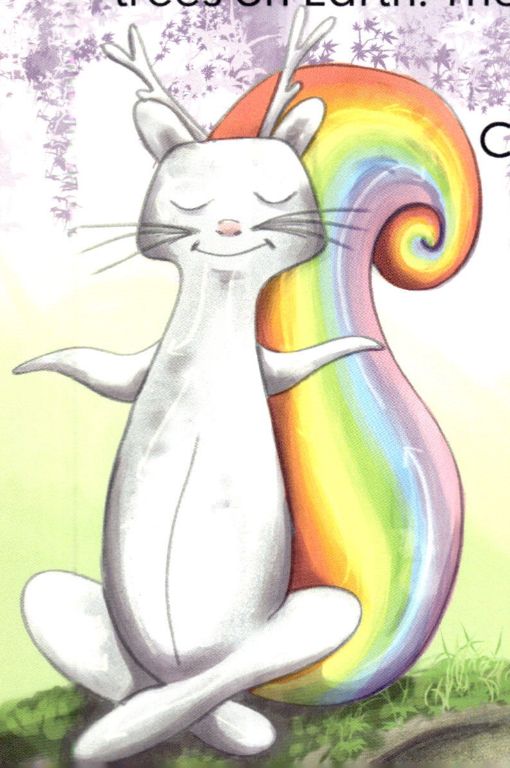

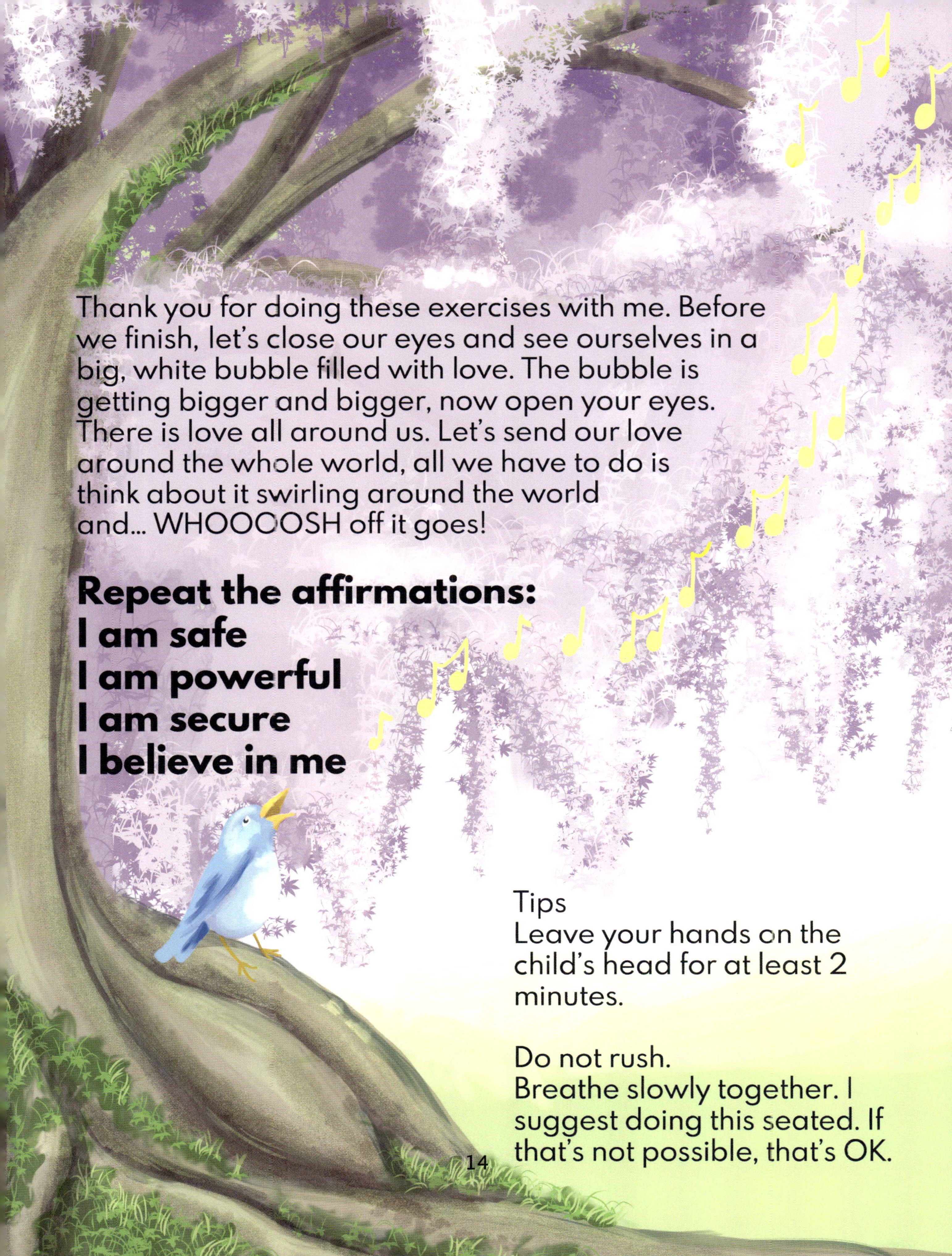

Thank you for doing these exercises with me. Before we finish, let's close our eyes and see ourselves in a big, white bubble filled with love. The bubble is getting bigger and bigger, now open your eyes. There is love all around us. Let's send our love around the whole world, all we have to do is think about it swirling around the world and... WHOOOOSH off it goes!

Repeat the affirmations:
I am safe
I am powerful
I am secure
I believe in me

Tips
Leave your hands on the child's head for at least 2 minutes.

Do not rush.
Breathe slowly together. I suggest doing this seated. If that's not possible, that's OK.

Heart to Head

We can open and close our eyes anytime we want. Can I put my hands on your head? Now, you put yours on mine. Do you see any colour? How does your head feel today? Is it busy, fuzzy, happy or sad? I think we should send lots of love to our heads. Imagine that the love from your heart flows down your arms and into my head. I will send lots of love to your head now.

Can you feel my love flowing into your head? Wow! You are very good at sending love, my head can feel your beautiful, warm heart energy.

Thank you so much.

It's important that we send our head lots of love, it's busy all day long thinking and doing things. The love you're sending me is helping me feel safe, calm and relaxed.
How do you feel?

Even when I'm not with you, if your head ever becomes too busy, I want you to put your own hands on your heart and breathe deep into your heart. Then after five deep breaths, place your hands on your head and send it lots of love.

Feel your head fill up with the love you have sent yourself. You will feel calmer.

Thank you for doing these exercises with me. Before we finish, let's close our eyes and see ourselves in a big, white bubble filled with love. The bubble is getting bigger and bigger, now open your eyes. There is love all around us. Let's send our love around the whole world, all we have to do is think about it swirling around the world and...
WHOOOOSH off it goes! The more we do this, the stronger our love becomes.

Repeat the affirmations:
I am loved
I am happy
I am kind to myself
I am open to all the abundance of the universe

Tips
Make it fun together.
Talk about how your intentions are so powerful.
Sip a glass of water that you have both infused with good energy after the session.
You can do this anywhere and anytime.

Communication

colour. Imagine that colour is a
it is in our throats. Can you see it?
ings that were great about your day
asn't so good? Let's put our hands
down on the page.
Let all the bad things and thoughts from today flow out from you onto the page. Feel them flowing down your arms and out of your hands onto the page. Together let's blow them away. Take a big breath in and blow out like you are trying to blow out a big candle. All those bad thoughts are blowing away!

See all the bad thoughts like seeds floating away to soon grow into beautiful flowers of love and peace. I wonder what colour the flowers will be, what colour do you think they will be?

Now your body has lots of space for wonderful things to happen. The bad thoughts have gone, do you feel lighter? Like a feather?

I feel ____.

Let's think about the good things which happened today and the good things we can fill ourselves up with tomorrow...

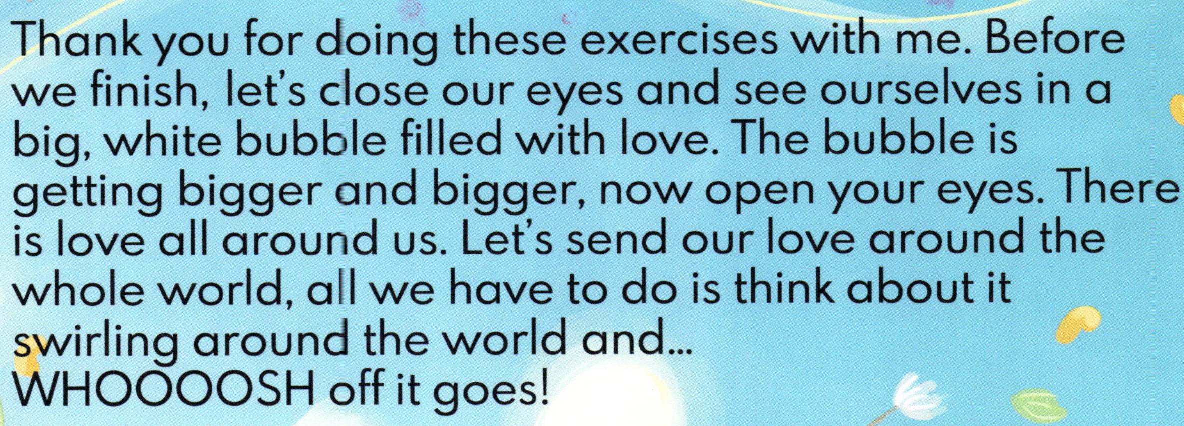

Thank you for doing these exercises with me. Before we finish, let's close our eyes and see ourselves in a big, white bubble filled with love. The bubble is getting bigger and bigger, now open your eyes. There is love all around us. Let's send our love around the whole world, all we have to do is think about it swirling around the world and...
WHOOOOSH off it goes!

Repeat the affirmations:
I am honest
I trust myself
I speak my truth
I can express myself with ease

Tips
Let the child know that when they are in the bath or washing their face and hands in the morning or night, that they can do this exercise.
The more they practice it the more powerful it becomes. You can do this anywhere and anytime.

Heart Emotions

Let's take a big deep breath into our hearts. How is your heart feeling today?
Mine is _______.

We aren't always happy and filled with joy, that's OK. What makes you super happy? What makes you sad? Sometimes we can feel happy and sad at the same time too! Emotions can be big or small. Sometimes they can make us feel a bit overwhelmed.

I'm going to show you how to help your heart to cope with emotions. Let's practice now and remember, you can do this anytime you need it. Close your eyes. Imagine a big, white jug. It's filled up to the very top with golden sparkling water. This is magical water.

See the water pouring slowly into your heart.

This water is cleansing away anything that doesn't make you feel happy and loved.
All those difficult emotions are being cleansed.
The magical water is washing away all your worries and sadness. Can you see them flowing off your heart and being washed away? See your heart shine and sparkle now! You can do this anytime and anywhere when you feel your heart has become a little dull. Just close your eyes and see the magical, golden water cleanse your heart.

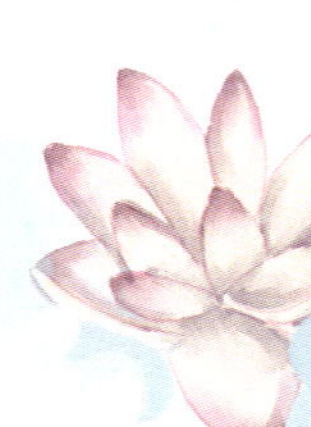

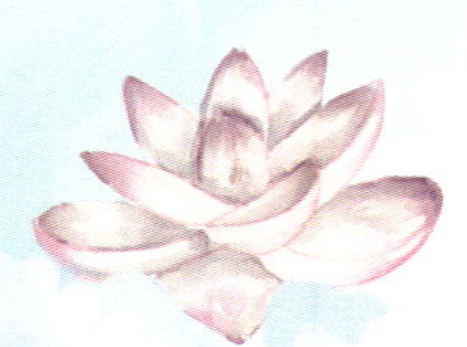

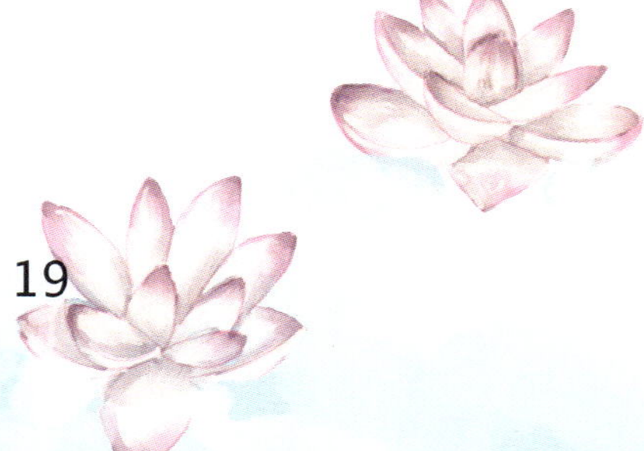

Thank you for doing these exercises with me. Before we finish, let's close our eyes and see ourselves in a big, white bubble filled with love. The bubble is getting bigger and bigger, now open your eyes. There is love all around us. Let's send our love around the whole world, all we have to do is think about it swirling around the world and...
WHOOOOSH off it goes!

Repeat the affirmations:
I am happy with life
I am feeling complete peace
I trust my feelings

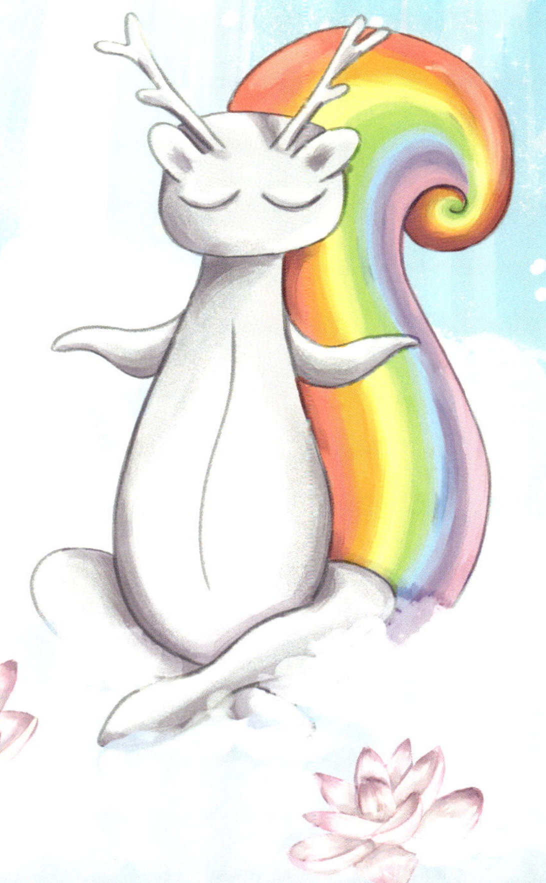

Tips
Pick a night each week and write down all the things you are grateful for and put them somewhere safe. At the end of the month read them all together.
Sit in a comfortable position for this exercise.

Tummy Love

Let's focus on our tummies. Sometimes when I am worried, I feel like there is a butterfly flying around inside my belly. What makes you worry sometimes? How does that make you feel?

Let's pretend that you have shrunk down really small, popped inside your own belly and caught the butterfly carefully with a net. Now put that butterfly in a jar, can you see it inside the jar?
Isn't it beautiful?
What colour are its wings?
My butterfly's wings are ____.

But butterflies can't live in jars, we need to help the butterfly get out. Imagine you have gone back to your normal size and you are holding the butterfly in the jar. To set the butterfly free, we have to talk about any worries you might have. Tell me your worries.

What made you feel like you have a butterfly inside? As you're telling me your worries, the jar is getting lighter and lighter until... PUFF it disappears and the butterfly is free to fly away! How does your tummy feel now? Mine is all calm like a lake on a sunny day.

We can still give our tummies love even when they don't feel too fluttery, we can share time together talking about the things that are on our minds and filling our hearts full of love for each other. I love sharing time with you like this.

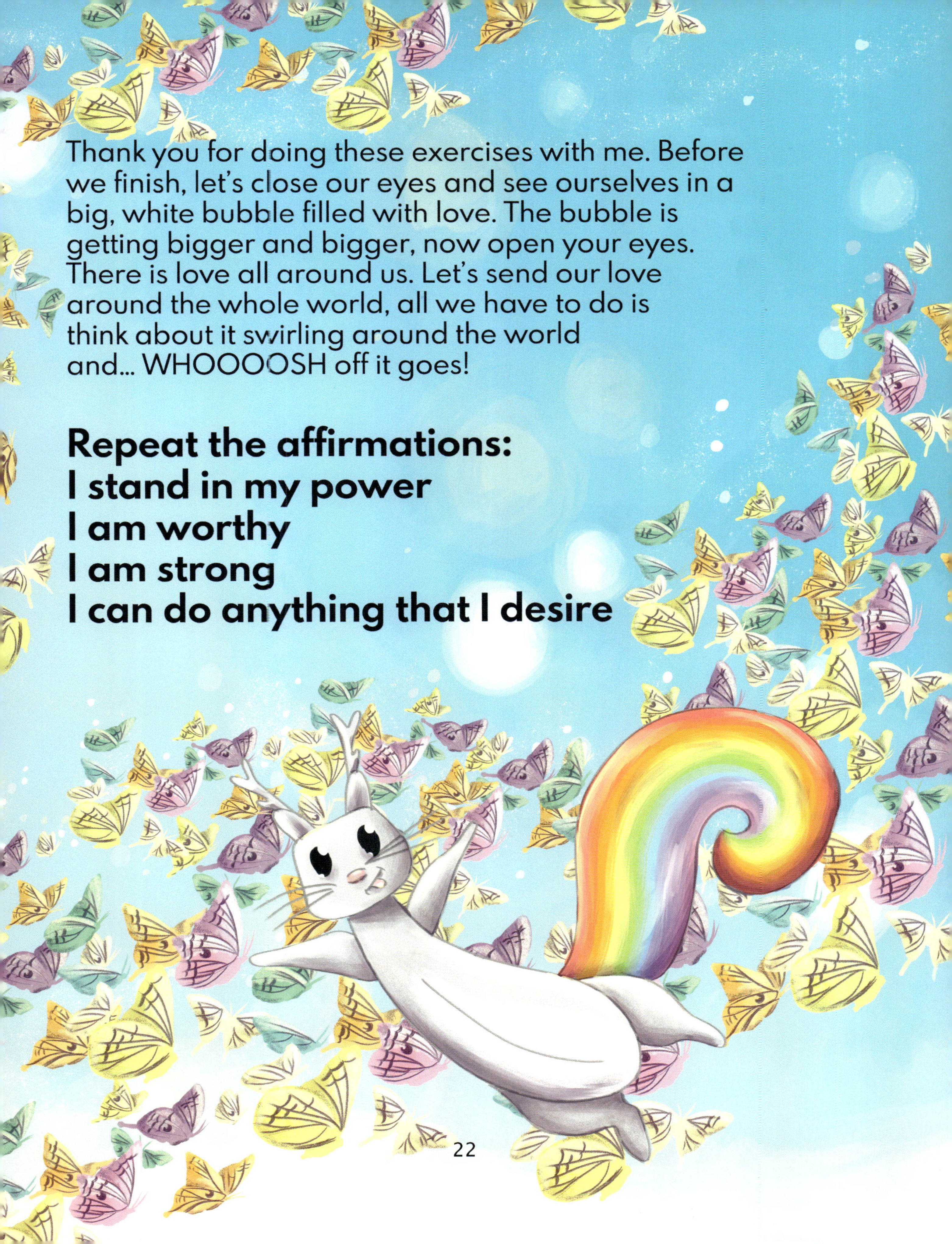

Thank you for doing these exercises with me. Before we finish, let's close our eyes and see ourselves in a big, white bubble filled with love. The bubble is getting bigger and bigger, now open your eyes. There is love all around us. Let's send our love around the whole world, all we have to do is think about it swirling around the world and... WHOOOOSH off it goes!

Repeat the affirmations:
I stand in my power
I am worthy
I am strong
I can do anything that I desire

Magical Journey

Bring your hands to just below your belly button. Take a deep breath into your hands. Let's try to see a door in our minds, can you see it? What colour is the door? My door is ____.

Let's open it and go inside. What do you see? Let's go on a magical journey. Where will we go? Space? An enchanted forest? Anywhere you want, you tell me. What will we do there? Tell me all about it.

I am so excited to be on this magical journey with you and spending time together.

It is time to go back through the door. See it closed now, just until our next magical trip together.

That was so much fun. I love going on magical trips with you.

Thank you for doing these exercises with me. Before we finish, let's close our eyes and see ourselves in a big, white bubble filled with love. The bubble is getting bigger and bigger, now open your eyes.
There is love all around us. Let's send our love around the whole world, all we have to do is think about it swirling around the world and...
WHOOOOSH off it goes!

Repeat the affirmations:
I am complete
I accept all my emotions
I feel clear and free
I am all that I need

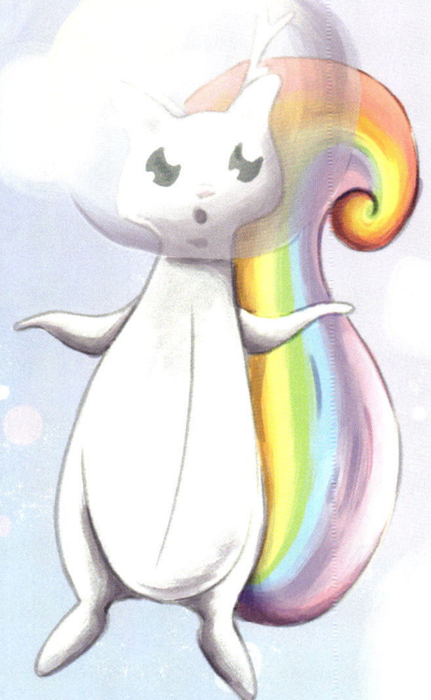

Tips
If possible this is a nice exercise to do lying down or seated. If the child gets lost for words, help them along the way.
Imagination work comes with practice and patience.
Enjoy the time together.

Red Cave

Put your hands on your hips, breathe all the way down to your hips. Imagine a red light going through your whole body all the way down into the centre of the Earth. I can see a beautiful red cave. Inside are magical gemstones and lots of different animals. Crystals and gemstones are very powerful and give off beautiful healing energy. I am excited to meet the animals, are you?

There is a strong fluffy bear here called Cherokee. Do you know that in some cultures they say we all have an animal that helps to look after us? I think Cherokee looks after you.
He is strong and brave, yet loving and soft.

If you ever feel afraid and unsure, close your eyes and call Cherokee. Imagine Cherokee giving you a big bear hug. Let's wrap our arms around each other and squeeze tight. That feels so nice. You are strong and brave like the bear. There are many other wonderful animals that we can learn about together. Next time we visit the Red Cave we can meet some of the other animals. I feel nice and calm now.

How do you feel?
It's lovely to think that we have a beautiful animal that cares for us.

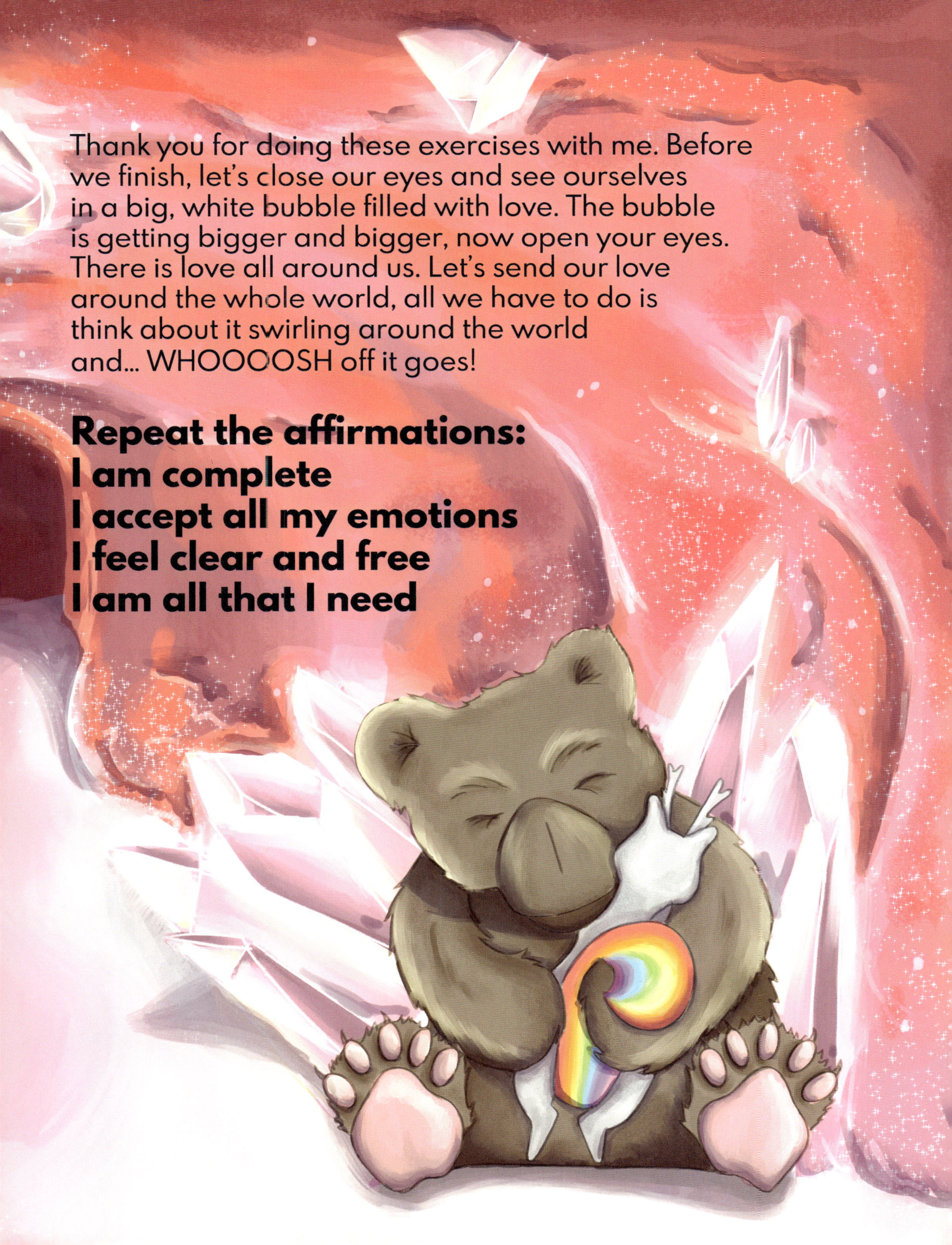

Thank you for doing these exercises with me. Before we finish, let's close our eyes and see ourselves in a big, white bubble filled with love. The bubble is getting bigger and bigger, now open your eyes. There is love all around us. Let's send our love around the whole world, all we have to do is think about it swirling around the world and... WHOOOOSH off it goes!

Repeat the affirmations:
I am complete
I accept all my emotions
I feel clear and free
I am all that I need

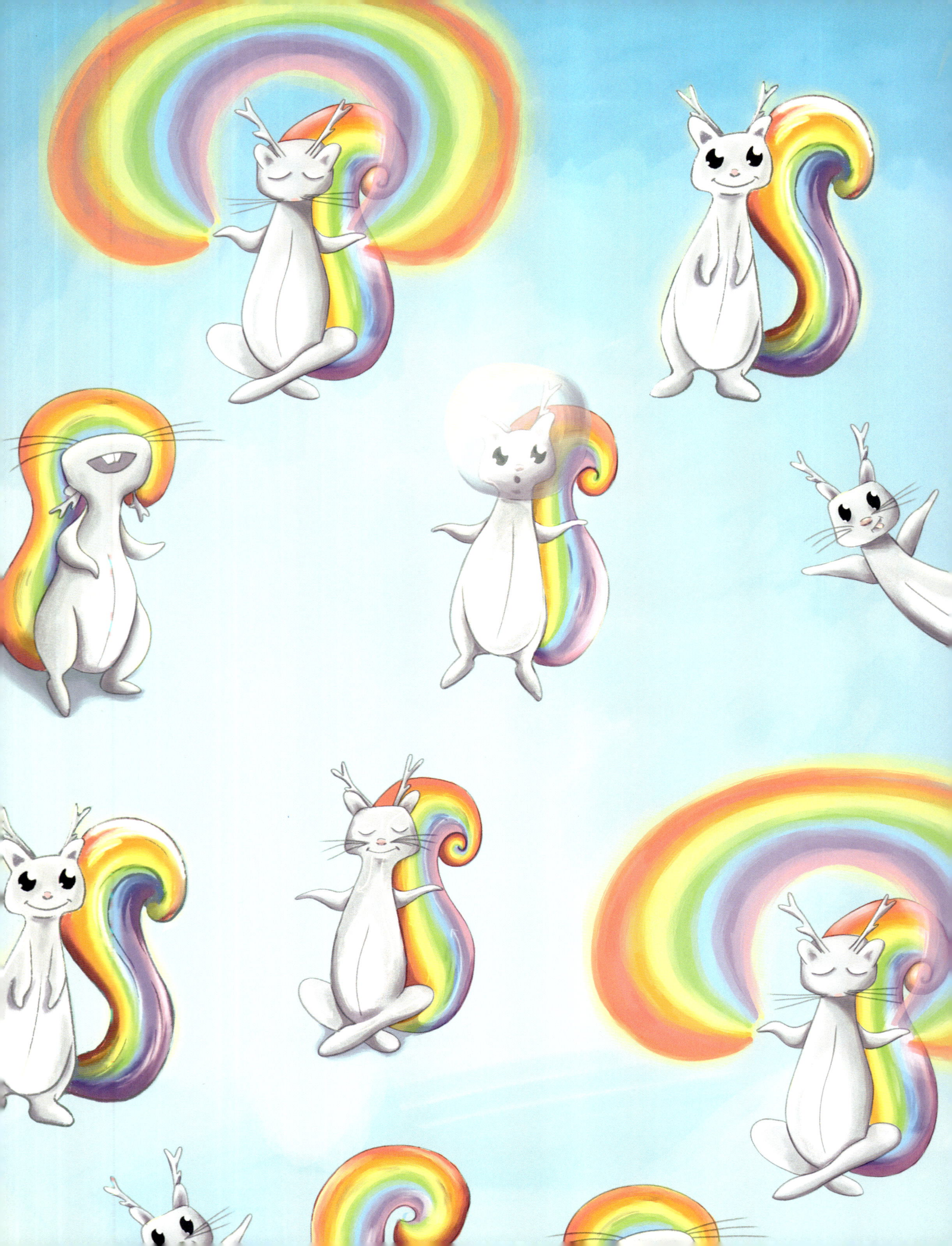

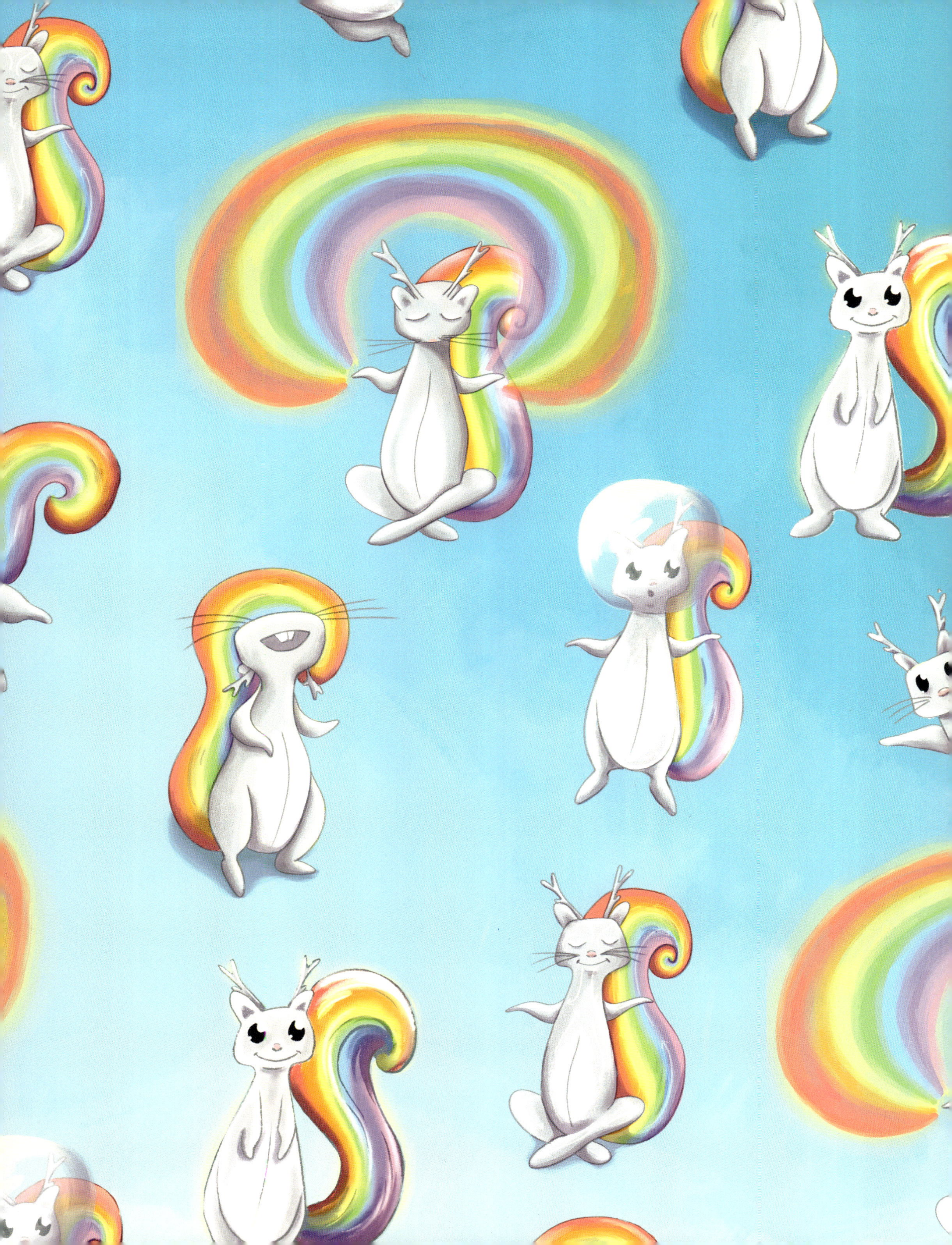

Liz Reilly is a writer, and author of the new book, A time for us. In her writing she hopes to introduce ways in which adults and children can connect, have fun and express there emotions in a fun and safe way.

She has worked with children with additional needs in schools in Ireland and on a one to one basis. She has taught children and adults yoga and also provides reiki healing sessions for adults and children.

Liz has one son Hugo who inspired the writing of this book, who is on the autism spectrum.

When not teaching or writing she loves to walk the local wexford beaches with her dogs, teddy and Foggy. She also has a magical black cat Luna who is so playful and fun.
To stay connected and updated on upcoming material and events you can follow and contact Liz at,

Insta @bhakti_healing
Facebook Bhakti Healing
Website Bhaktihealing.ie
Email info@bhaktihealing.ie

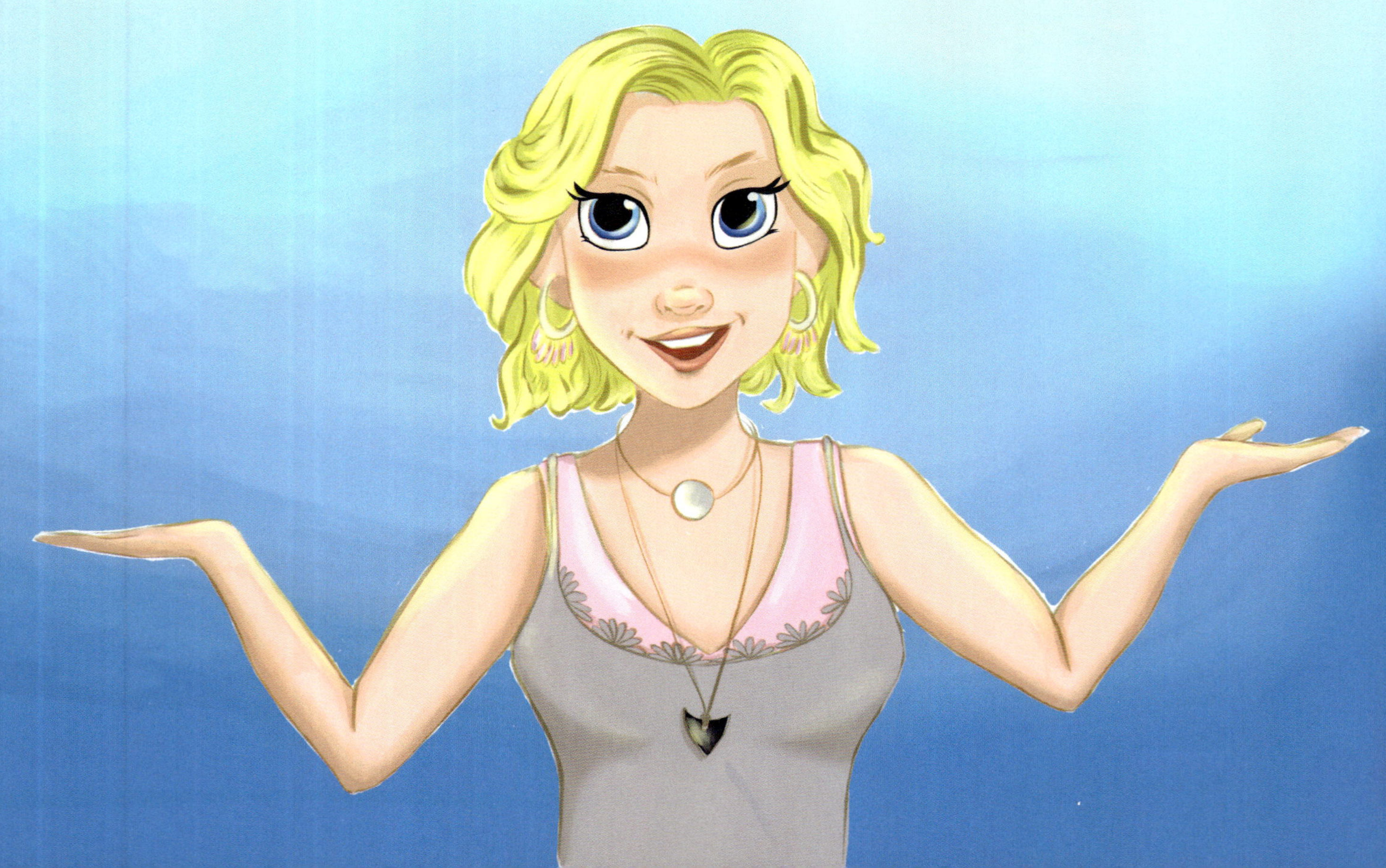

Printed in Poland
by Amazon Fulfillment
Poland Sp. z o.o., Wrocław

65841560R00021